FALL ASLEEP LIKE A BABY EVERY NIGHT

SLEEP EXPERT'S GUIDE TO FALLING INTO DEEP SLUMBER WITH EASE AND RISING WITH ENERGY

SOHAIB MANZOOR NATNOO

Made with ♥ on the Notion Press Platform
www.notionpress.com

All Praise and Thanks belong to Allah, the Almighty, with whose permission this effort resulted in something tangible.

I am also so grateful to my grandfather who never misses a chance in supporting me through words of prayer, my mother who kills her happiness for mine, and my father who goes way above and beyond to provide me with everything that I need, my uncle and aunt who are always there to encourage me to expand my boundaries, and both my sisters who keep showing their love for me.

And my heartfelt thanks to two of my beloved friends, Shoaib Akhter and Mehran Farooq, especially Mehran Farooq who supported me when I was about to crumble. May Allah grant both of them the best of both worlds!

Also, I want to take a moment to express my gratitude and appreciation to my teacher, guide, support system, and best friend. This person has been with me through thick and thin and has been a constant source of support, encouragement, and love.

Without this person's unwavering belief in me and my abilities, this book would not be possible. My best friend has been my sounding board and my cheerleader throughout this entire process, and I am forever grateful.

So, to my best friend, thank you. Thank you for always being there for me, for pushing me to be my best, and for helping me bring this book to life. You are an incredible human being and I am so lucky to have you in my life.

Contents

Acknowledgements

In today's fast-paced world, people have a lot on their plate, whether it's work, social commitments, family obligations, or personal interests. This often leaves little time for self-care, including getting enough quality sleep. Many people are constantly on the go, rushing from one activity to the next, and may not prioritize their sleep as much as they should. This can result in a variety of sleep-related problems, from difficulty falling asleep or staying asleep to feeling tired and irritable during the day.

"Fall Asleep like a Baby Every Night" addresses these issues by providing a brief and to-the-point solution to sleep-related problems. The book is designed to be easily digestible and practical so that busy individuals can quickly learn about the importance of sleep, the science behind it, and the various factors that can impact it. The book then goes on to offer simple, yet effective, solutions to common sleep problems, such as creating a relaxing sleep environment, establishing a consistent sleep schedule, and adopting good sleep hygiene habits.

By presenting this information in a concise and accessible manner, "Fall Asleep like a Baby Every Night" aims to make it easier for individuals to prioritize their sleep and take steps to improve its quality. This can have a significant impact on their overall health and well-being, allowing them to perform at their best and enjoy life to the fullest.

Preface

Do you struggle with sleep? Do you lay in bed at night, counting sheep or listening to white noise, just hoping to fall asleep? If so, you're not alone. Millions of people all over the world suffer from sleep difficulties, and it can be a frustrating and exhausting experience. But there is hope.

This book, "Fall Asleep like a Baby Every Night," is a go-to guide for anyone looking to improve their sleep. It contains bite-sized chapters, stuffed with a value that you can read in a minute or so, but have the potential to change your sleep life forever. Whether you're a busy professional, a parent, or just someone who wants to sleep better, this book has something for you.

Each chapter is designed to be quick and easy to read, yet packed with valuable tips and techniques that you can use right away to improve your sleep. You'll learn about the importance of Prayer, sleep hygiene, how to create a sleep-conducive environment, and how to relax and calm your mind before bed. You'll also discover the power of prayer and how it can help you sleep better.

So, if you're ready to say goodbye to restless nights and hello to a good night's sleep, then this book is for you. Let's start your journey to better sleep, and fall asleep like a baby every night!

Foreword

I am thrilled to introduce this book, which I wrote as a 20-year-old student, and it's my first book. As a student, I know firsthand the importance of getting enough sleep, especially during times of intense academic pressure. Balancing the demands of school, work, and social life can be challenging, but I firmly believe that taking care of our physical and mental health is crucial to achieving our goals and living our best lives.

This book is a result of my personal experience and research into the topic of sleep. I've struggled with sleep issues in the past, and I've learned various techniques and strategies that have helped me achieve a better night's sleep. In this book, I share these insights with you, so that you too can fall asleep like a baby every night.

Through the pages of this book, you'll learn about various factors that can affect your sleep, including your sleep environment, diet, exercise, and stress levels. I provide practical tips for creating a relaxing bedtime routine and managing sleep disorders, such as insomnia and sleep apnea.

I am excited to share this book with you, and I hope that the strategies and techniques presented within will help you achieve a better night's sleep. By improving your sleep, you can improve your physical and mental health, enhance your academic and personal performance, and increase your overall sense of well-being. Thank you for reading, and I wish you all the best on your journey towards better sleep.

Attention

As you read through this book, you'll notice that each chapter ends with a section called "Takeaway." This section is designed for you to do an active recall of what you've learned and to have something tangible to work on after reading each chapter. The empty space provided after the "Takeaway" section is for you to jot down notes or insights that you want to remember and implement in your sleep routine.

Remember, the ultimate goal of this book is to help you fall asleep like a baby every night, and to do that, it's important to take an active role in your sleep journey. The tips and techniques outlined in this book are meant to be applied and practiced, not just read and forget.

So, as you read through each chapter, take some time to reflect on what you've learned and make a plan for how you'll incorporate the new information into your sleep routine. By doing this, you'll have a better chance of making a lasting change and finally enjoying the benefits of a good night's sleep.

Note: 'Expert' in the title is used casually to describe my ability to sleep well. It does not point to any of my professional designations.

ONE

THE POWER OF PRAYER

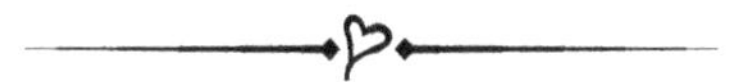

Once upon a time, there was a woman named Sarah who struggled with sleep every night. No matter what she did, she just couldn't seem to fall asleep easily or stay asleep for more than a few hours at a time. Frustrated and tired, Sarah tried everything she could think of to improve her sleep. She read books, tried relaxation techniques, and even saw a doctor. But nothing seemed to work.

One day, Sarah's friend told her about the power of prayer and suggested that she ask God for help. At first, Sarah was skeptical. She didn't see how praying could help her sleep better. But her friend was persistent, and Sarah decided to give it a try. That night, before she went to bed, Sarah prayed and asked God to help her sleep better. And to her surprise, she slept like a baby!

No matter how many sleep tips and techniques Sarah tried, they never seemed to be effective until she started asking God for His help. The truth is that the biggest weapon you have to improve your sleep is your ability to ask Him. When you pray and ask God to help you sleep better, you tap into a power that is beyond anything else you can do.

Many people struggle with sleep difficulties because they don't understand the importance of asking God for help. They may be doing everything right - practicing good sleep hygiene, using relaxation techniques, and following all the other tips for a good night's sleep - but without His blessing, their efforts will not yield the desired results. This is because 99 percent of people want to do well, but fail because God does not allow them to do so.

So, if you want to get ahead and achieve a peaceful and restful sleep, start by asking God for His help. Pray for His guidance and support, and ask Him to bless your efforts to improve your sleep. When you do this, you open yourself up to His power and allow Him to work in your life. With His help, you will find that your sleep improves, and you will be able to enjoy the many benefits that come from a good night's rest.

In conclusion, the power of prayer should not be underestimated when it comes to improving your sleep. Remember, no matter how much you try to do it on your own, without God's blessing, your efforts will fall short. So, make it a habit to ask God for His help, and you will be amazed at the difference it can make in your sleep.

KEY TAKEAWAY

TWO

INTRODUCTION TO SLEEP AND ITS IMPORTANCE

Welcome to "Fall Asleep Like a Baby Every Night". I am thrilled that you're joining me on this journey to better sleep. Before we dive into the practical tips and tricks to get you sleeping like a baby, let's start with the basics.

In this chapter, we'll cover the topic of sleep and its importance. You might be surprised to learn how crucial sleep is for our physical and mental health. We'll review why it's essential and what happens in our bodies when we sleep. So, grab a cup of tea, and let's get started!

First off, let's talk about why sleep is important. Our bodies need sleep to recharge and repair. During sleep, our bodies produce hormones and proteins that help to restore and refresh our muscles, tissues, and cells. Additionally, sleep is crucial for our mental health. During sleep, our brains process and consolidate memories, regulate emotions, and solve problems. Without proper sleep, we can feel fatigued, and irritable, and struggle to focus and be productive during the day.

Now, let's talk about what happens in our bodies during sleep. There are two main stages of sleep: Non-REM (Rapid Eye Movement) and REM. Non-REM sleep is the first stage of sleep and is divided into three stages. During this stage, our bodies relax and repair. Our heart rate and breathing slow down, and our muscles become more relaxed. In the second stage of Non-REM sleep, our bodies become even more relaxed, and our brain waves slow down. Finally, in the third stage, we enter a deep sleep, and our bodies start repairing and restoring tissues and cells.

The second stage of sleep is REM sleep. This stage is crucial for our mental health as it's during this stage that our brains process and consolidate memories, regulate emotions, and solve problems. During REM sleep, our eyes move rapidly, and our brain activity increases. This stage typically lasts for about an hour and happens several times throughout the night.

In conclusion, sleep is essential for our physical and mental health. Without proper sleep, we can feel fatigued, and irritable, and struggle to focus and be productive during the day. By understanding what happens in our bodies during sleep, we can appreciate the importance of getting enough quality sleep each night.

Now that we've covered the basics, it's time to dive into how we can improve our sleep. In the next chapters, we'll cover topics such as sleep disorders, sleep environments, sleep hygiene, and more. Get ready to say goodbye to sleepless nights and hello to sweet dreams!

KEY TAKEAWAY

THREE

UNDERSTANDING SLEEP DISORDER

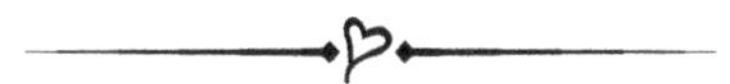

In this chapter, we'll be discussing sleep disorders and how they can impact our sleep quality. Sleep disorders are more common than you might think, and they can range from minor issues like difficulty falling asleep to more serious conditions like sleep apnea. Understanding sleep disorders is the first step to overcoming them and getting a good night's sleep every night.

Let's start by discussing the most common sleep disorders. Insomnia is one of the most common sleep disorders and is characterized

by difficulty falling asleep or staying asleep. People with insomnia often feel tired and irritable during the day and have trouble concentrating. Another common sleep disorder is sleep apnea. Sleep apnea is a serious condition in which a person stops breathing several times a night, causing them to wake up frequently. People with sleep apnea may feel excessively tired during the day and may have trouble concentrating.

Another sleep disorder is restless leg syndrome, which is characterized by an irresistible urge to move the legs while trying to sleep. This can make it difficult to fall asleep or stay asleep and can lead to restless nights. Narcolepsy is another sleep disorder, characterized by excessive daytime sleepiness and sudden episodes of sleep. People with

narcolepsy may find it difficult to stay awake during the day and may fall asleep at inappropriate times.

It's also important to note that some medical conditions, such as depression and anxiety, can cause sleep disorders. People with these conditions may find it difficult to fall asleep or stay asleep, leading to a cycle of sleep deprivation that can make their symptoms worse.

Now that we've discussed the most common sleep disorders, let's talk about how they can be treated. The treatment for a sleep disorder depends on the specific condition, but there are several methods that can be effective. For example, people with insomnia may benefit from practicing good sleep hygiene, such as creating a relaxing bedtime routine and avoiding screens before bedtime.

People with sleep apnea may benefit from using a continuous positive airway pressure (CPAP) machine or undergoing surgery to correct the underlying cause of the disorder. People with restless leg syndrome may benefit from taking medications to relieve their symptoms.

In conclusion, sleep disorders are more common than you might think, and they can range from minor issues like difficulty falling asleep to more serious conditions like sleep apnea. Understanding sleep disorders is the first step to overcoming them and getting a good night's sleep every night. If you think you might have a sleep disorder, it's important to speak with your doctor. They can help you.

determine the cause of your symptoms and provide you with the best treatment options.

In the next chapter, we'll dive into the science of sleep and what happens in our bodies during the night. Until then, sweet dreams!

TAKEAWAY

FOUR
THE SCIENCE OF DEEP SLEEP

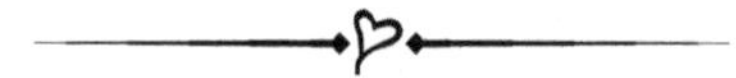

Now let's talk about the chemicals that regulate sleep. There are several key hormones and neurotransmitters that play a role in regulating sleep. Melatonin is a hormone that is produced by the pineal gland in response to darkness and helps to regulate our sleep-wake cycle. Serotonin is a neurotransmitter that is involved in regulating our mood and is also thought to play a role in regulating sleep. Adenosine is a chemical that accumulates in the brain throughout the day and signals to the brain that it's time to sleep.

In addition to these key chemicals, our sleep-wake cycle is also regulated by a part of the brain called the hypothalamus. The hypothalamus controls our circadian rhythms or the internal biological clock that regulates our sleep-wake cycle. Our circadian rhythm is influenced by light exposure and other environmental factors.

Now that we've discussed the different stages of sleep and the chemicals that regulate sleep, let's talk about why sleep is so important for our health. Sleep is essential for physical and mental health. During sleep, our bodies repair and rejuvenate themselves. Sleep also helps to boost our immune system and protect against illness. Additionally, sleep is important for our mental health and well-being. Sleep helps to regulate our mood, reduce stress, and improve our ability to think and concentrate.

One of the most important processes that occur during sleep is memory consolidation. Memory consolidation is the process by which our brain organizes and stabilizes new memories so that they can be easily retrieved later. During sleep, especially during slow-wave sleep, the brain replays experiences from the day and integrates them into our long-term memory. This helps to strengthen the connections between neurons, making it easier to recall the information later on.

Another important process that occurs during sleep is the regulation of hormones. Sleep plays a crucial role in the regulation of hormones such as cortisol, insulin, and growth hormone.Cortisol is a stress hormone that is involved in regulating our metabolism and immune system. Insulin is a hormone that regulates our blood sugar levels. Growth hormone is involved in the growth and repair of tissues and muscles. When we don't get enough sleep, the levels of these hormones can become disrupted, which can lead to a range of health problems, including obesity, type 2 diabetes, and weakened immunity.

Sleep also plays an important role in regulating our mood. Research has shown that lack of sleep can lead to depression, anxiety, and irritability. During sleep, our brains process and regulate our emotions. When we don't get enough sleep, our emotional regulation can become disrupted, leading to mood swings and emotional instability.

Finally, let's talk about the role of sleep in overall health. Sleep plays a crucial role in maintaining our physical health. During sleep, our bodies repair and regenerate damaged tissues. Sleep also boosts our immune system, helping to protect against illness. In addition, sleep helps to regulate our metabolism, maintain a healthy weight, and lower the risk of developing chronic health conditions such as heart disease and stroke.

In conclusion, the science of sleep is a complex and fascinating field of study. From memory consolidation to hormone regulation to overall health, sleep plays a crucial role in our lives. By understanding the deep science of sleep, we can better appreciate the importance of getting a good night's sleep every night.

In the next chapter, we'll discuss tips and tricks for improving your sleep quality. So get ready to dream the night away!

FIVE

THE SLEEP ENVIRONMENT

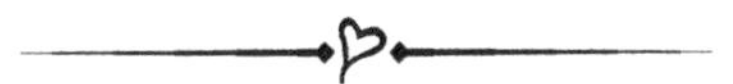

Let's talk about the importance of creating a sleep-friendly environment! Your sleep environment can have a big impact on the quality of your sleep, so it's important to pay attention to the details.

First and foremost, let's talk about your bed. A comfortable mattress and pillows are key to getting a good night's sleep. Make sure your bed is supportive and comfortable, and consider investing in quality bedding that will keep you cool and cozy all night long.

The temperature of your sleep environment is also important. Our bodies naturally cool down at night to signal to our brains that it's time to sleep. A room that is too warm can disrupt this process and make it difficult to fall asleep. Aim to keep your sleep environment at a temperature of around 65-70 degrees Fahrenheit.

Light is another important factor to consider in your sleep environment. Light signals to our brains whether it's time to be awake or asleep. When it's dark, our bodies produce melatonin, a hormone that makes us feel sleepy.

Exposure to light in the evening can disrupt the production of melatonin and make it difficult to fall asleep. Consider using blackout curtains or an eye mask to block out any light from your sleep environment.

Noise can also be a problem in the sleep environment. Loud or persistent noises can make it difficult to fall asleep and stay asleep. Consider using earplugs or a white noise machine to help block out unwanted noise and create a peaceful sleep environment.

Finally, it's important to consider the layout and organization of your sleep environment. Make sure that your bed is positioned away from any sources of light or noise, and consider using a bedside table or lamp to keep your phone and other devices out of reach. This will help to reduce the temptation to check your phone or engage with screens before bed, which can disrupt sleep patterns and make it difficult to fall asleep.

In conclusion, the sleep environment is a crucial component of getting a good night's sleep. By paying attention to the details and creating a sleep-friendly environment, you can improve the quality of your sleep and enjoy all of the benefits that come with getting a good night's sleep. From comfortable bedding to a peaceful and organized sleep environment, these small changes can make a big difference in the quality of your sleep.

TAKEAWAY

SIX

SLEEP HYGIENE

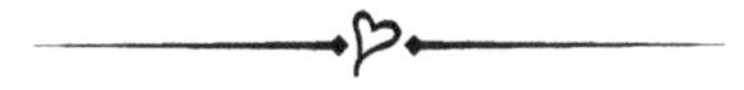

Let's talk about the importance of sleep hygiene! Sleep hygiene refers to the habits and practices that promote healthy sleep. By following good sleep hygiene, you can improve the quality of your sleep and enjoy all of the benefits that come with getting a good night's sleep.

First and foremost, it's important to establish a consistent sleep schedule. Our bodies thrive on routine, and going to bed and waking up at the same time every day helps to regulate our internal sleep clock and improve the quality of our sleep.

Next, let's talk about the importance of a relaxing bedtime routine. This can include anything from taking a warm bath or shower to reading a book or practicing relaxation techniques like deep breathing or meditation. The goal of a bedtime routine is to help you wind down and prepare your body and mind for sleep.

It's also important to avoid stimulants before bed. This includes things like caffeine and cocaine, which can disrupt the quality of your sleep. Try to avoid these substances in the hours leading up to bedtime, and if you do consume caffeine, make sure to do so in moderation.

Physical activity is also important for good sleep hygiene. Regular exercise has been shown to improve sleep quality, so try to get regular physical activity during the day, but avoid vigorous exercise in the hours leading up to bedtime as this can be stimulating and make it difficult to fall asleep.

Finally, let's talk about the importance of avoiding screens before bed. The blue light emitted by devices like phones, laptops, and televisions can disrupt the production of melatonin and make it difficult to fall asleep. Try to avoid screens for at least an hour before bedtime, and consider using a blue light filter on your devices if necessary.

In conclusion, sleep hygiene is an essential component of getting a good night's sleep. By following good sleep hygiene practices, you can improve the quality of your sleep, regulate your internal sleep clock, and enjoy all of the benefits that come with getting a good night's sleep. From establishing a consistent sleep schedule to avoiding screens before bed, these small changes can make a big difference in the quality of your sleep.

TAKEAWAY

SEVEN

SLEEP AND LIFESTYLE

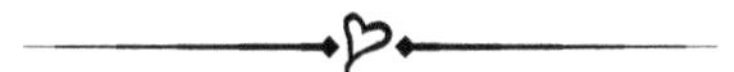

Let's talk about the impact of lifestyle on sleep! Your daily habits and routines can have a big impact on the quality of your sleep, so it's important to be mindful of the lifestyle choices you make.

First, let's talk about stress. Chronic stress can make it difficult to fall asleep and stay asleep, so it's important to find healthy ways to manage stress in your life. This can include things like exercise, meditation, or talking to a therapist.

Next, let's talk about diet. Eating a healthy and balanced diet can help to regulate your internal sleep clock and improve the quality of your sleep. Try to avoid heavy or greasy meals close to bedtime, and consider incorporating foods that are high in magnesium, such as almonds or leafy greens, into your diet, as magnesium has been shown to improve sleep quality.

Alcohol and caffeine can also have a big impact on sleep, as we discussed earlier. Try to limit your caffeine intake, especially in the hours leading up to bedtime, as this can disrupt the quality of your sleep.

Physical activity is also important for good sleep. Regular exercise has been shown to improve sleep quality, so try to get regular physical activity during the day, but avoid vigorous exercise in the hours leading up to bedtime as this can be stimulating and make it difficult to fall asleep.

Finally, let's talk about the importance of creating a sleep-friendly environment. This includes things like having a comfortable bed, regulating the temperature of your sleep environment, and minimizing exposure to light and noise. By creating a sleep-friendly environment, you can improve the quality of your sleep and enjoy all of the benefits that come with getting a good night's sleep.

In conclusion, your lifestyle can have a big impact on the quality of your sleep. By being mindful of the choices you make and incorporating healthy habits into your life, you can improve the quality of your sleep, regulate your internal sleep clock, and enjoy all of the benefits that come with getting a good night's sleep. From managing stress to creating a sleep-friendly environment, these small changes can make a big difference in the quality of your sleep.

TAKEAWAY

EIGHT

NATURAL SLEEP AIDS

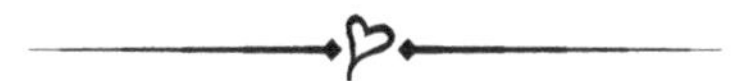

Let's talk about natural sleep aids! If you're looking for ways to improve the quality of your sleep without relying on medication, there are a number of natural sleep aids that you can try.

First, let's talk about herbal remedies. Herbs like valerian root, chamomile, and passionflower have been used for centuries to promote sleep and reduce anxiety. These herbs can be taken in supplement form or as tea before bed. Just be sure to talk to your doctor before trying any new herbal remedies, as some herbs can interact with other medications you may be taking.

Next, let's talk about aromatherapy. Essential oils like lavender, bergamot, and cedarwood have been shown to promote relaxation and improve sleep quality. You can try diffusing these oils in your sleep environment or using a pillow spray to help you relax before bed.

Magnesium is another natural sleep aid that you can try. Magnesium has been shown to improve sleep quality, and it's also important for overall health. You can find magnesium in foods like almonds, leafy greens, and avocados, or you can try taking a magnesium supplement before bed.

Finally, let's talk about sleep-promoting activities. Activities like meditation/ and deep breathing can help to reduce stress and promote relaxation, making it easier to fall asleep and stay asleep. Try incorporating these activities into your bedtime routine to help you wind down and prepare for sleep.

In conclusion, there are much natural sleep aids that you can try if you're looking to improve the quality of your sleep. From herbal remedies to sleep-promoting activities, these natural remedies can help you get the restful sleep you need to feel your best. Just be sure to talk to your doctor before trying any new remedies, and remember that a healthy lifestyle, good sleep hygiene, and a sleep-friendly environment are all important components of getting a good night's sleep.

TAKEAWAY

NINE
OVER-THE-COUNTER SLEEP AIDS

Let's talk about over-the-counter sleep aids! If you're having trouble falling asleep or staying asleep, there are a number of over-the-counter sleep aids that you can try.

First, let's talk about antihistamines. Antihistamines like diphenhydramine (found in products like Benadryl) have a sedative effect and can help you fall asleep. Just be aware that these products can cause next-day drowsiness, so they should only be used as a short-term solution.

Next, let's talk about melatonin. Melatonin is a hormone that regulates sleep, and taking a melatonin supplement can help to regulate your internal sleep clock and improve the quality of your sleep. Melatonin supplements are available over-the-counter and can be found in various forms, including tablets, gummies, and liquids.

Herbal remedies, such as valerian root, chamomile, and passionflower, are also available over the counter in supplement form. These remedies can help to promote sleep and reduce anxiety, but be sure to talk to your doctor before trying any new remedies, as they can interact with other medications you may be taking.

It's important to keep in mind that over-the-counter sleep aids are not a long-term solution for sleep problems. They should only be used as a short-term solution to help you get through a period of disrupted sleep. A healthy lifestyle, good sleep hygiene, and a sleep-friendly environment are all important components of getting a good night's sleep, so be sure to focus on these things as well.

In conclusion, over-the-counter sleep aids can be a helpful short-term solution if you're having trouble falling asleep or staying asleep. Just be aware of the potential side effects and be sure to talk to your doctor before trying any new remedies. And remember, a healthy lifestyle, good sleep hygiene, and a sleep-friendly environment are all important components of getting a good night's sleep, so don't neglect these things as you work to improve your sleep.

TAKEAWAY

TEN

SLEEP AND TECHNOLOGY

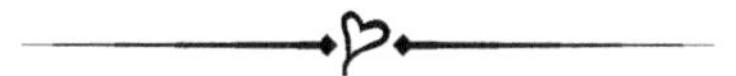

Let's talk about sleep and technology! With the increasing use of technology in our daily lives, it's important to understand how our devices and screens can affect our sleep.

First, let's talk about the blue light that's emitted from our screens. Blue light is known to suppress the production of melatonin, which is a hormone that regulates sleep. So, if you're using your phone, tablet, or computer an hour or two before bed, you may be disrupting your body's ability to produce melatonin and prepare for sleep.

To combat this effect, you can try using a blue light-blocking screen or app on your device, or you can simply avoid using screens an hour or two before bed. If you must use your device before bed, try using a warm light setting or using the device with a red light filter.

Another way technology can impact our sleep is by disrupting our sleep environment. For example, if you're using your phone as an alarm clock, it's easy to get distracted by notifications or emails, and this can disrupt your sleep and make it difficult to fall back asleep. To avoid this, try using a traditional alarm clock or a sleep-focused alarm app that will only play calming sounds and won't disrupt your sleep with notifications or emails.

Finally, let's talk about the impact of social media and technology on our mental health and stress levels. Spending too much time on social media can increase feelings of stress, anxiety, and depression, and these feelings can in turn impact the quality of our sleep. To avoid this, try to limit your use of social media and other technology before bed, and instead focus on relaxing activities like reading a book, taking a bath, or practicing meditation.

In conclusion, it's important to be mindful of how technology is impacting your sleep. From the blue light emitted from our screens to the impact of social media on our mental health, there are a number of ways that technology can disrupt our sleep. By making simple changes to our technology habits and taking steps to create a sleep-friendly environment, we can improve the quality of our sleep and feel more rested and refreshed.

TAKEAWAY

ELEVEN

SLEEP AND MENTAL HEALTH

Let's talk about the connection between sleep and mental health. Our sleep and mental health are interconnected in many ways, and it's important to understand this connection in order to improve both.

First, let's talk about how poor sleep can impact our mental health. Lack of sleep can increase feelings of anxiety, depression, and stress, and it can also make it more difficult to manage symptoms of mental health conditions like anxiety or depression. When we don't get enough sleep, we may also have trouble concentrating, making decisions, and regulating our emotions, which can make it more difficult to cope with daily stressors.

Now, let's talk about how our mental health can impact our sleep. If we're feeling anxious, stressed, or depressed, it can be difficult to fall asleep and stay asleep. Negative thoughts and feelings can keep us up at night, making it difficult to get the rest we need to function at our best.

So, what can we do to improve the connection between our sleep and mental health? Here are a few tips:

- Practice good sleep hygiene: This includes things like going to bed and waking up at the same time every day, creating a relaxing bedtime routine, and avoiding screens an hour or two before bed.
- Manage stress: There are many effective stress-management techniques, including exercise, meditation, and deep breathing. Find what works for you and make it a part of your daily routine.
- Talk to your doctor: If you're struggling with poor sleep and mental health, talk to your doctor. They can help you determine the cause of your symptoms and provide you with appropriate treatment options.

In conclusion, our sleep and mental health are closely connected, and taking steps to improve our sleep can have a positive impact on our mental health and well-being. By practicing good sleep hygiene, managing stress, and talking to our doctor, we can improve the quality of our sleep and feel more rested and refreshed.

TAKEAWAY

TWELVE
THE END

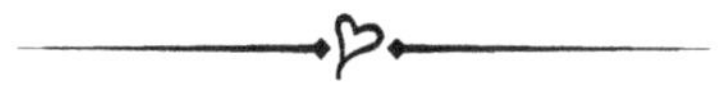

Well, we've come to the end of our journey! I hope you've found "Fall Asleep Like a Baby Every Night" to be informative and helpful. Throughout this book, we've explored the importance of sleep, the science of sleep, and the many factors that can impact our sleep, including sleep disorders, sleep environment, sleep hygiene, lifestyle, and technology.

As we've seen, getting enough quality sleep is crucial for our overall health and well-being. Whether we're students, busy professionals, or retirees, we all need sleep to help us perform at our best and feel our best. And, by making a few simple changes to our sleep environment, sleep habits, and lifestyle, we can improve the quality of our sleep and feel more rested and refreshed each day.

So, as I wrap up this book, I want to encourage you to keep exploring the world of sleep. Keep learning, keep trying new things, and keep striving to find the sleep habits and routines that work best for you. Remember, the journey to better sleep starts with you, and with a little effort and patience, you can fall asleep like a baby every night.

Thank you for joining me on this journey, and I wish you sweet dreams!

What Changes Will You Make In Your Sleep Routine After Reading This Book?

Author's Note

I'm delighted that you have been enjoying my work - Fall Asleep Like a Baby Every Night.

To stay in touch with me, please head over to Instagram, LinkedIn, and YouTube to check me out. I'd truly be overjoyed if you'd share your experiences with this guide and how it has benefited your slumber quality with these platforms or any other ones regularly used by you. Your appreciation is invaluable to me.

Thank you for taking the time to read my book and for considering following me on social media. I look forward to connecting with you and hearing your thoughts on the book.

Wishing you sweet dreams!

Socials

Instagram: Sohaib Natnoo
LinkedIn: Sohaib Natnoo
YouTube: Sohaib Natnoo

Some Fantastic Books To Read

- THE QURAN (TRANSLATION BY HAFIZ NAZAR)
- THE 100: A RANKING OF THE MOST INFLUENTIAL PERSONS IN HISTORY BY MICHEAL H HART
- RECLAIM YOUR HEART BY YASIM MOGAHED
- REVIVE YOUR HEART BY NOUMAN ALI KHAN
- DIVINE SPEECH BY NOUMAN ALI KHAN
- DISEASES OF THE HEART AND THEIR CURE BY IMAM IBN TAYTMIYYAH
- THE 5 AM CLUB BY ROBIN SHARMA
- THE FORTY RULES OF LOVE BY ELIF SHAFAK
- THE ALCHEMIST BY PAULO COELHO
- ATOMIC HABITS BY JAMES CLEAR
- DEEP WORK BY CARL NEWPORT
-

Printed by Libri Plureos GmbH in Hamburg,
Germany